Medicinal Plants

The Ultimate Guide to Medical Plants that Heal

Table of Contents

Introduction 6

The Various Medicinal Plants, It's Uses and Benefits...8

    Aloe Vera.. 8

    Alfalfa 9

    Arnica montana.. 10

    Euphorbia hirta 12

    Momordica charantia... 14

    Vitex agnus-castus... 16

    Dong Quai 17

    Sambucus nigra 18

    St. John's Wort 20

    White Willow 22

    Turmeric... 24

    Valerian 26

    Tea Tree Oil 27

    Tripterygium wilfordii 28

    Summer Savory 30

    Passion Flower 32

    Nimtree 34

    Moringa oleifera 36

- Kava Kava 38
- Mitragyna speciosa 40
- Equisetum 42
- Hoodia 44
- Henna 46
- Fenugreek 48

Conclusion 50

Introduction

Medicinal plants have been in used since time immemorial from Chinese herbal medicine to the Egyptians, and Ayurvedic medicine of India to name a few. Today, medicinal plants are still used under the umbrella of alternative medicine, which is likewise known as traditional medicine. According to modern standards of medicine, medicinal plants are pushed as alternative medicine because its practice is not based solely on the scientific method.

Although, many proponents of herbalism have pointed out that current pharmaceutical drugs are compounds derived from plants—however, the difference lies on the substantial studies produced by these pharmaceuticals to prove its efficacy and safety. This then fires up medicinal plant's proponents retort that there is no big money to be had if traditional medicine is studied because everybody has easy access to these plants. Likely, this could be the driving reason behind why scientific studies are not conducted on the efficacy and safety of herbal medicine. Thus, herbal medicine can only rely on anecdotal evidence plus ancient and cultural use of herbal plants—which for a lot of people is good enough. But even then, there are several independent studies that have shown and proven that certain medicinal plants are not only effective but are also safer than its pharmaceutical counterpart.

Without Further ado, let's not waste time and space on discussing medicinal plants as a whole. Let's get busy getting to know each medicinal plant's quality and benefit to get you started in creating your own medicinal plant concoctions.

The Various Medicinal Plants, It's Uses and Benefits

Aloe Vera

Aloe Vera is a widely distributed plant worldwide and hence has various medicinal applications. This medicinal plant is well-known to help various skin problems and contains soothing, healing and rejuvenating properties.

Benefits

- The aloe Vera gel or extract is helpful for providing relief for minor sores, frostbite, sunburns and even hemorrhoids.
- It can decrease plaques caused by psoriasis.

How to Use

It is easy to use aloe Vera, just get one leaf, remove the spines and squeeze out the gel. Apply the gel on the affected part, spread and leave on.

Alfalfa

Scientifically known as *Medicago sativa*, alfalfa is also called as Lucerne in New Zealand, South Africa and the UK.

Benefits

- It is known as a blood purifier and helps in reduction of cholesterol and high blood pressure.
- A known antidote when it comes to menstrual cramps and discomfort during menopause.
- It helps in increasing breast milk supply and even allays morning sickness.
- Alfalfa is also believed to help boost the immune system and the digestive tract.

How to Use

Alfalfa does not have a strong flavor and is quite bland so adding it to your usual meal will not change the flavor of the dish, but instead will increase its nutrient value. If using alfalfa as a medicinal plant eat it just as you would any salad green. Dried forms of alfalfa are also rich in protein and can easily be crushed and grounded to a powder form and added to any dish.

Arnica montana

Arnica montana is the scientific name of a beautiful flowering plant that is native to the Carpathians, Southern Scandinavia and Southern Iberia. It is also referred to as mountain arnica, mountain tobacco, wolf's bane, leopard's bane, and Wolfesgelega (German for wolf's eye).

Benefits

- It is useful for general muscle and joint pain.
- Provides relief for arthritis that has been triggered by seasonal change.
- It is especially beneficial for muscle swelling or spasms from sports activity, muscle soreness, sprains and bruises.

How to Use

Arnica is available as a salve, pill, cream, ointment and tincture. When looking to use arnica, go for topical applications. Rub the tincture or ointments onto injured area and make sure that skin is not broken. Never apply arnica on wounds or broken skin because it is toxic when taken internally unless it is in the form of a pill.

You can also use arnica as a compress. Do this by mixing a pint of purified water and a tbsp. of arnica and mix. Dip in a gauze pad, slightly wring to remove excess solution and apply compress onto bruised area or arthritic joint. You can change compress every 4 to 6 hours until bruise or pain is gone.

Euphorbia hirta

There are so many benefits that you can get from *Euphorbia hirta* that can make a person become skeptical about its real use. But, let me tell you a firsthand experience of a dear colleague of mine about this wonderful weed. Yes, *Euphorbia hirta* is a considered a weed in the Philippines and grows just about anywhere. *Euphorbia hirta* is known under a lot of names like tawa-tawa, gatas-gatas, hairy spurge, asthma plant, Koko kahiki, dudeli and so much more.

Benefits

- In the Philippines, tawa-tawa is a number one medicinal plant that's effective in bringing down high fever.
- Tawa-tawa has also been helpful and effective in fighting off Dengue Fever in the Philippines. Dengue fever is a common occurrence in the area especially during the rainy months of June to November. Dengue fever is a mosquito borne hemorrhagic illness where platelets can go extremely low and where the sickness has no cure except for rehydration. A lot of anecdotal evidence has pointed to this weed's efficacy in fighting off the disease.

- Other countries like India have pointed out that dudeli has been used in Ayurvedic treatment for digestive problems, respiratory ailments and female disorders.

How to Use

To help relieve high fever or fight off dengue fever or even increase your platelet count, just boil 2 cups of water to 1 plant stalk that's at least 6-inches long. First, properly clean the tawa-tawa plant stalk, discard the roots and wash thoroughly. Place in a pot with water and bring to a boil. Boil for just a minute, turn off fire and let it cool. You can add sugar to make it more pleasant to the taste and let the patient drink the tea, just as you would water until fever is gone. It is best to drink this tea for no more than one week straight at a time.

Momordica charantia

It is also known as balsam-pear, bitter squash, bitter gourd, bitter melon, ampalaya and so much more. Charantia is best known as a bitter vegetable and is used in a lot of Asian diseases.

Benefits

- One of the top and amazing benefits of charantia as a modern medicinal plant is its capability to pull down blood glucose levels. And because of this property, patients are also cautioned in checking their blood sugar levels because of the risk of suffering from low blood sugar.
- In Indian traditional medicine, this medicinal plant is also used to help relieve rheumatism, gout, ulcer, wounds, skin diseases, respiratory problems, cough, as a laxative and many others.

How to Use

Basically, charantia can be used as an ingredient in many Asian dishes. It can be pickled and used as an appetizing side dish. It is also cooked along with other vegetables and eaten. The bitter gourd leaves can also be eaten and you will still reap the same effects.

There are also commercially available charantia tea and capsules. The teas, you can drink it once or twice a day. As for the charantia capsules, it helps in controlling blood sugar levels and must be consumed according to manufacturer's instructions.

Vitex agnus-castus

This is a flowering plant that is commonly called as vitex, Monk's Pepper, Abraham's balm, Chasteberry or Chaste Tree. It has been used in Africa as part of their traditional medicine.

Benefits

- As a medicinal plant, vitex is used as a tonic for the reproductive system both for females and males. The leaves also provide the same property however to a lesser extent.
- In ancient times, vitex is believed to be an aphrodisiac thus its moniker "chaste tree."
- Currently in clinical studies, vitex has shown effectiveness in managing cyclical breast pain (mastalgia) and premenstrual syndrome (PMS).

How to Use

The berries, flowers or leaves of the vitex plant can be consumed as an elixir, tincture or decoction early in the morning, upon awakening as a 1:1 vitex extract and water. It is believed that it interacts with the hormonal circadian rhythms quite efficaciously.

Dong Quai

This Chines herb is known scientifically as Angelica sinensis. It is a native plant of Korea, Japan and China. A well-known and well-used medicinal plant, dong quai is also referred to as the female ginseng.

Benefits

- The dong quai medicinal plant is used to treat high blood pressure and cardiovascular conditions.
- It is also believe to be helpful in relieving menopausal vasomotor symptoms like hot flashes, thanks to its antispasmodic compound known as butylidenephthalide.
- The dong quai plant is also used to help relieve premenstrual cramps.

How to Use

Dong quai is now available in dried root, dried root slices, powder, dried leaf, decoctions and tinctures. All of these are available to be taken orally. Topical applications are also available for skin application. When drinking dong quai, just follow manufacturer's instructions.

Sambucus nigra

A flowering plant, the *Sambucus nigra* is known under a lot of names like: European black elderberry, European elderberry, European elder, black elder, elderberry or just elder.

Benefits

- It is beneficial for providing relief to occasional constipation because of its mild laxative and diuretic properties.
- The elderflower also contains antiseptic properties and works well as a mouth rinse.
- The elderflower can also be applied topically to help relieve swelling and pain related to arthritis. It is also capable of stopping bleeding when applied directly on the wound.
- It is also a great immune system booster because of its capability to kill virus and bacteria.
- The elder is commonly used to fight respiratory problems like sinus infections, flu and cold.

How to Use

Elderflowers should be cooked before using because it is toxic when eaten raw. You can simmer elderberry flowers for 15 minutes, strain and discard the flowers and drink the resulting tea. You can use 1 to 2 tbsps of the flowers per cup of water. You can drink the tea hot or cold, depending on your preference.

You can also find elderflower available in apothecaries either in concentrates, tinctures, tea bags, or dried and cut flowers. Use it according to specific manufacturer's instructions.

St. John's Wort

St. John's Wort is a well-known medicinal plant in the world of herbalism because of its anti-inflammatory, antibacterial and anti-depressant properties. Its scientific name is *Hypericum perforatum*. It is also referred to in many other names such as: Klamath weed, chase-devil, goatweed, rosin rose and Tipton's weed.

Benefits

- St. John's Wort is a widely accepted medicinal plant that effectively treats depression. In fact, in Germany it is frequently prescribed for moderate to mild depression in adolescents and children.
- It has anti-bacterial properties and has shown to be clinically effective against gram-positive bacteria.
- It can also be used as a topical remedy against muscle pain, burns, abrasions and wounds.
- Currently, St. John's Wort is being studied because of its possible usefulness as an effective treatment against alcoholism.

- Fresh evidence also points to St. John's Wort's efficacy in improving behavioral and physical symptoms related to premenstrual syndrome.
- Lastly, in a study conducted on rats St. John's Wort has shown to help alleviate age-related long-term memory loss.

How to Use

Since St. John's Wort is considered as a psychoactive drug, it is best to consult with an herbalist or physician first before using this medicinal plant. Then, follow doctor's recommendation.

If using *hypericum* to treat moderate to mild depression, 20-1,800 mg of St. John's Wort can be taken orally at least once to three times a day for 4 to 52 weeks.

For PMS (premenstrual syndrome), 300-900 mgs of St. John's Wort can be taken as per episode.

If using hypericum for wound healing, you can mix petroleum jelly with 20% St. John's Wort and apply on affected area of the skin at least once to three times a day for no more than two weeks.

White Willow

A type of medium sized deciduous tree, the white willow is known scientifically as Salix alba. It is a native plant of central and western Asia plus Europe. Did you know that salicin was isolated from this medicinal plant by the French pharmacist Henri Leroux in 1828? Yes, it is from the white willow that the active compound of aspirin and salicylic acid has been derived.

Benefits

- It helps reduce fever and is used as antipyretic, anti-inflammatory and as an analgesic.
- It helps prevent blood clot formation, strokes and heart attacks.
- Currently, studies have shown that salicin can be effective in fighting colorectal cancer.

How to Use

In earlier centuries, the willow bark is macerated in ethanol to create a tincture. However, it is now available is several forms and dosages like liquid, powder, capsules and tablets.

Remember that salicin is a potent compound and can be toxic to the liver; therefore extreme caution should be put into place when using this medicinal plant.

Turmeric

More famous for being a spice, turmeric is part of the ginger family and is a native plant of southeast India. Its active ingredient is curcumin which is believed to have wide ranging effects on the body like antiviral, antibacterial, antitumor, antioxidant and anti-inflammatory activities.

Benefits

- In Ayurveda medicine, turmeric has long been used to treat a wide range of diseases like sprains, wounds, pains, aches, gastrointestinal system, pulmonary system and including the skin.
- It is topically applied to help heal wounds and sores because of its anti-microbial properties.
- It is ingested to treat liver problems and as a remedy for stomach problems too.
- It is even applied on the face to fight off acne because of its anti-microbial property.

How to Use

Turmeric can easily be bought in powdered form from any grocery store. For skin applications, you can apply the powder directly on the skin. If you want it easier to apply, you can make a paste out of it by adding water to form a paste. Then spread on affected skin.

Turmeric is also safe to consume and is delicious to boot. You can enjoy a lot of curry dishes to help treat your stomach or liver problems. Some even use a teaspoon of turmeric in a glass of milk daily.

Valerian

Another widely used medicinal plant, the valerian is a perennial flowering plant which is endemic to Asia and Europe. It is widely sought for its sleeping effects. it is one of the few medicinal plants that has been scientifically studied and scientifically proven to provide effective relief for certain health conditions.

Benefits

- Valerian is regarded as an herbal medicine that can substitute as a hypnotic drug. It is even used as a substitute for sedatives that help in treating specific anxiety disorders.
- Valerian has long been touted to help fight insomnia. According to the American Journal of Medicine, Valerian can help improve the quality of sleep without side effects.

How to Use

Valerian is now available as an over the counter supplement. To help treat insomnia, a healthy dose of 400 to 900 mgs of Valerian can be taken orally at least 30 minutes to two hours before sleeping.

Tea Tree Oil

Tea tree oil is an essential oil that comes from the *Melaleuca alternifolia* leaves, hence its other moniker of Melaleuca oil. Although tea tree oil has enjoyed propaganda for several years now as an effective ingredient in facial washes, but little do people know that it is toxic when ingested.

Benefits

- Tea tree oil has been proven to help fight and eradicate a lot of skin problems like: herpes, lice, acne, dandruff and other skin problems.

How to Use

Tea tree oil comes as a clear liquid in a small bottle. You can make a facial wash, toner or shampoo out of your tea tree essential oil by adding at least 15 drops of tea tree oil to a 100ml of your favorite facial wash, toner or shampoo. You can also make use of over the counter 10% tea tree oil creams to fight off toe nail fungal infections.

Tripterygium wilfordii

This medicinal plant is also known under a lot of names like: thunder duke vine, thunder god vine, raikoto or lei gong teng. It has been used in traditional Chinese herbal medications for centuries and is just beginning to come into the spotlight.

Benefits

- The lei gong teng medicinal plant is believed to be effective in providing temporary antifertility effect for males.
- It is also believed to contain an active compound that could prove useful is treating systemic lupus erythematosus, rheumatoid arthritis and other autoimmune disorders.
- In clinical studies, lei gong teng contains triptolide which is being investigated for its promise as an anti-tumor agent and as an immune-suppressing agent.
- Current studies is also pointing out two compounds found in lei gong teng , the quinone triterpene celastrol and triptolide which shows potential in eliminating and reducing pancreatic tumors in mice.

How to Use

It is recommended that use of thunder god vine extract of 180 to 570 mgs per day for up to 20 weeks can be consumed in treating rheumatoid arthritis.
As for children with kidney problems, 1mg per kg of body weight can be given daily for up to 20 weeks.

Thunder god vine also come in tinctures which can be topically applied on joins for no more than 5 to 6 times a day for relief of rheumatoid arthritis.

Summer Savory

Summer savory is a popular medicinal herb in Atlantic Canada. It is scientifically known as *Satureja hortensis* which is commonly used as an herb too. For medicinal purposes, its stems and leaves are used to heal a variety of illnesses.

Benefits

- Summer savory is used to treat sore throat and coughs.
- It is also believed to be helpful in treating intestinal disorders like loss of appetite, nausea, diarrhea, gas, indigestion, and cramps.
- For patients suffering from diabetes, they use summer savory to decrease their polydipsia or frequent thirst.
- There are also times when summer savory is used to increase sex drive or as an aphrodisiac.
- In the field of medicine, it is believed that compounds within this medicinal plant are potent against fungus and bacteria. It also contains chemicals that can decrease muscle spasms.

How to Use

If using for sore throat and cough, you can steep a tablespoon of fresh leaves of the summer savory in a ½ cup of hot water. Let it stand at least ten minutes or until cold enough for you to gargle. You can gargle a few mouthfuls and repeat at least 3 times a day.

If using for other illnesses, the flowering shoots are best used. It can be boiled to create a tea or dried to be stored and used in the near future. Either way, the flowering shoots of the summer savory have anti-flatulence, antiseptic and expectorant properties.

Passion Flower

Passion flower is also known as passion vines, *Passiflora incarnate*, maypop, or Passiflora—which is the genus name of the plant. Many species of the passiflora are found all over the globe and some are cultivated because of its beautiful flowers. It is in North America that Passiflora is considered as a medicinal plant. Long used by Native Americans, its roots and leaves are valued because of its analgesic properties.

Benefits

- The passion flower is found to be effective in treating epilepsy, hysteria and insomnia.
- In a scientific study conducted in 2001, the maypop is an effective treatment for generalized anxiety disorder with fewer short term side effects than oxazepam.

How to Use:

For treating illnesses, the dried leaves of the passion flower can be smoked. If wanting to treat epilepsy, hysteria and insomnia, dried or fresh leaves of this medicinal plant is used to make tea and drank once a day just before bed time.

Nimtree

Nimtree is known under a lot of names and these are: Indian Lilac, Neem and its scientific name is *Azadirachta indica*. The nimtree has been considered a medicinal plant in India for over centuries and is actually used in ayurvedic medicine.

Benefits

- The neem tree is used as an antiviral, antibacterial, antifungal and as an anthelmintic. This means that it is used to cure infections.
- This medicinal plant is also used as a sedative, contraceptive and as an antidiabetic.
- The neem tree is also planted to keep away disease carrying mosquitoes in tropical countries.
- Aside from the above, the neem leaves are also used to treat psoriasis, eczema and other skin diseases.
- The neem oil is also used to balance blood sugar levels, detoxify the blood and enhance liver function.

- Not only is neem oil used in treating health conditions but it is also used in India to make hair more beautiful and healthier.

How to Use

It is advised that only short term use of neem oil is safe. Use of neem oil on children is totally prohibited because it can be toxic.

For skin use, the fruit, root bark and stem of this medicinal plant are used as an astringent and tonic. You can apply neem directly to the affected part of the skin or head to treat skin ulcers, wounds, skin diseases and even head lice.

The neem seed and seed oil are used to treat intestinal worms, leprosy, birth control and abortion. Neem twigs are effective against diabetes, urinary disorders, low sperm levels, intestinal worms, and hemorrhoids.

Moringa oleifera

Moringa oleifera is the scientific name for benzoil tree, ben oil tree, horseradish tree, drumstick tree, murungai, malunggay and many others. This medicinal plant is commonly referred to as Moringa. This medicinal plant has been used in Southeast Asia for centuries to treat wounds. Currently, the world has begun to look at it in a different light because not only does it pack a lot of nutrients, it also contains a lot of health benefits with constant consumption.

Benefits

- It is rich in Vitamin C and is therefore an immune-boosting food.
- Used as an antiseptic and for wound care.
- Consumed to help breast feeding mothers increase their milk production.
- In Ayurvedic medicine, moringa leaves are consumed in order to control glucose levels and blood pressure.

How to Use

It is easy to use moringa leaves in helping you achieve optimum health. If you have a moringa plant in your backyard, you can crush the leaves until it is a dark green color and wet. Apply on to your wound and leave until the next application. You can change your moringa dressing at around three times a day or until wound has closed.

If using moringa to help increase lactation or control blood sugar or hypertension, you can eat use the leaves in soup based recipes and eat it daily or as many times as you like in a day. However, do remember that nutrients are lost when the leaves are cooked in very high fire at around 140°F. So, the proper way of cooking moringa is to cook your soup and any meat or fish in eat. When it is done, turn off the fire, add the moringa leaves, stir and let it sit for 3 minutes before serving.

There are already moringa supplements available in the market these days. You can use them if moringa is not available in your neighborhood. Just follow manufacturer's instructions when it comes to consumption.

Kava Kava

Kava kava or simply called as Kava is scientifically known as *Piper methysticum*. Other names of this medicinal plant are: sakau, yaqona, ava, wild cognac (waild koniak) and awa.

Benefits

- Kava kava is used to make a person relax without affecting mental clarity. Hence it is good for treating short term social anxiety.
- It is also used for its sedative and anesthetic effects.

How to Use

The traditional preparation of kava kava happens in many ways. The first method is the pounding of the roots of the kava plant. The second method is grinding the kava bark and root with a tiny bit of water. Then the resulting mush is added to cold water and drank as quickly as possible.

The third method is to chew the kava root or bark—and this provides the strongest effect. Kava is also available in prepared forms like dried, powdered and even pills.

Mitragyna speciosa

This medicinal plant belongs to the coffee family and is a native plant of Southeast Asia. The *Mitragyna speciosa* is also known as kratum and ketum.

Benefits

- It has psychoactive properties and helps uplift the mood in low doses.
- The ketum is also used to treat health problems.
- It is also used to manage pain in high doses.

How to Use

The kratom leaves can be chewed fresh to experience the effects of this medicinal plant. Usually, the stringy central vein of the leaf is removed prior to chewing. Kratom leaves can also be dried before chewing, but more people prefer to crush it into a powder when dried and add it to juices.

Tea can also be made from dried kratom leaves by steeping the leaves in hot water for around 10 minutes. Then the leaves are strained and discarded before it is sipped. Sometimes, to make it more palatable people add it to black tea or add honey to the kratom tea.

Equisetum

Equisetum is a genus of plants that has been living on earth for over a hundred million years. It is likewise known as puzzlegrass, snake grass or horsetail. *E. arvense* is a specific species of this medicinal plant that has been traced back to Roman and Greek medical sources which was served as an herbal remedy.

Benefits

- *E. arvense* is used to improve bone health, hair, and skin.
- It is also used to control weight.
- This medicinal plant is also used to invigorate your senses and well-being.
- In South America, *E. giganteum* is used to treat kidney disorders, bladder problems and urinary infections by acting as a diuretic; thereby it also helps in reducing swelling related to excess retention of fluids.
- Currently, studies have pointed to the possibility of horsetail in inhibiting cancer cell growth with its antioxidant properties.

How to Use

Horsetail is available in two different preparations and these are liquid preparation and dried herb. Horsetails are not recommended for us on children because it contains nicotine. For adults the standardized dosing are as follows: external compresses: 10 grams of herb per liter of water daily; tinctures should be on a ratio of 1:5 at 1 to 4 ml no more than three times a day; for herbal infusions like tea, 2 to 3 teaspoonful no more than 3 times a day. Add hot water on the herb and let it steep for no more than ten minutes and drink as directed. When taking horsetail preparations orally, it is highly recommended that you drink plenty of water in order to prevent dehydration because it is a potent diuretic.

Hoodia

Hoodia is a current favorite of weight loss proponents because of its appetite suppressing capabilities. This medicinal plant is endemic to South Africa and although it may look like a cactus, they are not related at all. Locally, it is known as the Queen of Namib, xhoba and Bushman's Hat. Scientifically, Hoodia is the genus name and under it, it has several species. However, the most common medicinal plant being used today is the *Hoodia gordonii*.

Benefits

- It can suppress the appetite which is used by locals during long hunting trips in a sparsely vegetated area to suppress appetite and stave off hunger.

How to Use

The world has taken great notice of this medicinal plant because of its possibility in helping people with weight problems to reach their desired weight. Hoodia is now available over the counter as health supplements. However, it is highly cautioned that before taking in hoodia, please talk with your doctor first especially if you have a bleeding disorder, heart disease, diabetes and/or an eating disorder.

Henna

Henna is widely known as a dye used in temporary tattoos. However, henna is also a plant where the henna dye comes from. It is also known as the Egyptian privet, mignonette tree, henna tree, hina or through its scientific name of *Lawsonia inermis*. In ayurvedic and unani medicines, this medicinal plant's seeds and barks are used in traditional healing practices.

Benefits

- The henna oil can be applied topically on the affected part of the skin to treat burns, fungal infections, scabies and eczema.
- The henna bark is used in treating enlargement of spleen and liver, likewise symptoms of jaundice too.
- The henna oil from its flowers is used for relieving muscular pains. While the seed oil is used in regulating menstruation and as a deodorizer too.
- The henna extracts have been shown in current clinical studies to possess ultraviolet light screening activity, antifungal and antibacterial properties.

- Henna oil is also believed to help healthy hair growth.

How to Use

For headaches, joint pain and skin problems henna oil can be applied topically to the affected part. Henna oil is also used on hair to help prevent appearance of gray hairs.

For liver problems, the henna bark is used. Thirty to fifty grams of henna decoction can be taken to cure liver problems.

To help cure baldness, in a pan heat 250 grams of mustard oil. Once hot add 50 to 60 grams of henna leaves and sauté for 5 minutes on low fire. Filter the oil and discard leaves. Massage oil on to scalp regularly until healthy hair grows.

Fenugreek

Fenugreek is best known for being a spice hailing from the Indian subcontinent and the Mediterranean. But little do people know that this plant has been used and eaten even before biblical times. Plus, fenugreek is also considered a medicinal plant because of the various health benefits that you can gain from it aside from its curative effects too.

Benefits

- Historically, fenugreek is used to treat reproductive problems like reduction of menstrual pain, for breast enlargement, treatment of hormonal disorders, for inducing labor and others.
- In China and India, fenugreek is used to treat bronchitis, sore throat, acid reflux, asthma, arthritis, and skin problems like boils, rashes and wounds.
- Aside from treating illnesses, fenugreek is also used in enhancing male potency and libido.

How to Use

For skin problems, ground one tablespoon of fenugreek seeds into a powder. In a medium bowl, mix in with a cup of warm water. Dip a clean cloth and apply cloth like a poultice on the affected part.

If you want to treat acid reflux, stomach problems, cough and sore throat simply add a teaspoon of fenugreek seeds on your food. You can also swallow the teaspoon of seeds before eating your meal with juice or water.

If you want to naturally enhance the size of your breast, then use fenugreek as a part of your daily diet. The traditional consumption is up to 3 grams of fenugreek seeds per day.

Conclusion

This list is by no means an exhaustive list of all the medicinal plants of the world. The list of medicinal plants that I have given you above is varied in terms of its uses and efficacy so that whatever ailment your household may face, you have some arsenal for each and every disease.

I hope that you will have an effective time using these medicinal plants against common ailments.

Copyright © 2015. All rights reserved.

Except as permitted under the United States Copyright Act of 1976, reproduction or utilization of this work in any form or by any electronic, mechanical, or other means, now known or hereafter invented, including xerography, photocopying, and recording, and in any information storage and retrieval system, is forbidden without written permission.

The ideas, concepts, and opinions expressed in this book are intended to be used for educational and reference purposes only. Author and publisher claim no responsibility to any person or entity for any liability, loss, or damage caused or alleged to be caused directly or indirectly as a result of the use, application, or interpretation of the material in this book.

Printed in Great Britain
by Amazon